# NO MORE BILE REFLUX

## HOW TO CURE YOUR BILE REFLUX AND BILE GASTRITIS NATURALLY WITHOUT MEDICATIONS

### PAUL HIGGINS

ISBN-13: 978-1976331206 | eBook ISBN: B075K2V91P

Printed in the United States of America

First Edition: September 2017

Second Edition: May 2020

# TABLE OF CONTENTS

# INTRODUCTION

*Is this the first time you've experienced symptoms of bile reflux, heartburn or bile gastritis, or have you been a victim for life? Whatever your answer is, you've come to the right place.*

Thousands —even millions— of people around the world are in the same situation, suffering daily with bile reflux, gastritis and heartburn. The sad thing is that most of them don't receive the right treatment, and those who are being treated by conventional medicine are caught in a circle of medications that merely relieve symptoms without offering a long-term solution.

Regardless of whether you have experienced the symptoms of bile reflux or gastritis or have witnessed the trauma that causes gastritis in someone you know or care about, you're definitely not alone. According to the *American Gastroenterology Association,* approximately 2.9 million people are affected by gastritis within the United States, and about 300,000 new cases are reported every year. However, the truth is that many physiological, mechanical and dietary factors can contribute to the development of bile reflux and bile gastritis.

I suffered with this condition for several years and visited many gastroenterologists, and none of the medications they prescribed me helped at all, and many even made me feel worse—not to mention all the money I spent on procedures, blood tests, therapies and drugs.

It was really frustrating to pay for an expensive test or procedure only to conclude that everything was fine. All that, plus the side effects some of the medications caused, made me feel depressed and hopeless about someday being normal again.

I'm sure you understand how it feels, not being able to do the things you want, like working, studying, hanging out with friends, and eating or drinking the foods and beverages you love. It's really more than a "stomach problem"; it affects your entire life.

After several years of visiting doctors and spending a lot of money, I finally decided to do things on my own. Day and night, I researched bile reflux. During that time, I learned how the digestive system works (including the physiology of gastrointestinal secretions), how and why bile reflux happens, what bile is, what its function is and why it can cause problems in the stomach.

And in this guide, I will reveal you the truth about bile reflux, including everything you need to know about this problem and what you can do to overcome it. This guide is NOT intended to replace the complete and accurate diagnosis of your doctor. However, I have vast experience in the subject and have conducted in-depth research, exploring the work of many experts in digestive subjects. Thus, I've written this guide so that anyone —especially those suffering from bile reflux and bile gastritis— can read and understand it.

As you read the following pages, you'll better understand this condition and how it affects your body. You'll discover alternatives to conventional treatments in the form of suggestions for a more holistic approach towards healing —an approach that is more conducive to the natural forms of the body.

Sun Tzu said in the book *The Art of War*: "If you know the enemy and you know yourself, you do not have to fear the outcome of a hundred battles." In other words, knowing why your bile reflux happens will help you feel more prepared to take it on with a clear and effective strategy, such as the one described in this guide.

# CHAPTER 1

## KNOWING THE PROBLEM

Before starting to treat the problem, it's important that you know what is responsible for the problem. This includes knowing the symptoms it produces, the possible causes and all those things that will help you have a better understanding and knowledge of the problem. So, let's start learning more about what's responsible for the whole problem – nothing more than a fluid produced in the liver, known as "bile".

### What is Bile and How Does it Work?

Bile is produced in the liver and stored in the gallbladder. When you ingest foods (especially fatty ones), the liver begins to produce bile, which is stored in the gallbladder while digestion is carried out. Once the food has been broken down into small particles in the stomach, bile is released into the first portion of the small intestine, called duodenum, through the sphincter of Oddi so that it can mix with the food when it leaves the stomach. In cases in which the gallbladder has been removed by cholecystectomy (surgery), the liver continues to create bile to aid in digestion.

The release of bile is due to a complicated system that works in a synchronized way, as well as to hormonally controlled feedback, which involves different hormones. The digestive system is very complicated; some of the hormones it involves are gastrin, secretin, cholecystokinin, motilin and ghrelin... and there are probably more to be discovered.

Gastrin is a hormone secreted into the bloodstream by the stomach. Its release is triggered by the presence of certain foods in the stomach (particularly peptides and amino acids). This hormone causes stomach acid to be secreted into the stomach through the parietal cells and is inhibited when the stomach pH falls below 3. Gastrin also interacts with many other hormones, relaxes the lower esophageal sphincter, strengthens antral contractions against the pylorus, maintains pyloric sphincter tone and (also via other hormones) triggers the production of bile. Apparently, this system hasn't been understood completely, as it seems as though many doctors don't know much about how this works.

Most of us know what gastric juices are and how they work, but bile is a completely different fluid that the digestive system uses to emulsify the fats we ingest through foods. It also serves to neutralize the gastric juices or the acid chyme in the duodenum so that it doesn't irritate the intestinal walls.

## Appearance of Bile

Bile may vary somewhat in appearance. Its color ranges from dark green to yellowish brown. It has a bitter taste that can be experienced if bile is present in the esophagus. Generally, bile ascends the esophagus during gastroesophageal reflux. If this is the case, the problem should be solved, because this situation can lead to other complications.

Bile is not acidic or produced in the stomach, although this may be hard to believe because the burning sensation it causes makes you think otherwise. However, the truth is that it isn't acidic. Bile is actually ALKALINE and consists of water, acids, biliary salts, mucus, pigments, cholesterol and some inorganic salts.

## Breaking Down Fats

The purpose of bile is to break down or emulsify the fats we take in through our diet. After food has spent time churning within the stomach, it passes into the small intestine and there gets mixed with bile.

Small amounts of fat are surrounded by bile to prevent the formation of large globules of fat. Once this happens, an enzyme from the pancreas makes its way between the bile salts to digest parts of the fat and to get to the nucleus or center of the digested food.

This is extremely important because the fats must be broken down before they can pass through the walls of the intestine to be used by the body. If this process is not carried out, the fats simply go through the body without being digested, which on many occasions (depending on the amount of fat ingested) will result in diarrhea.

## Other Purposes of Bile

In addition to this digestive function, bile performs other important tasks. For example, it helps clean the blood. When red cells are recycled by the liver, they create a waste product called bilirubin. In large quantities, this substance can be toxic for the body; bile helps eliminate it.

Another of the "cleaning" functions of bile is to destroy dangerous microbes that may enter the body along with food. Also, as I said at the beginning of this chapter, bile can also help neutralize gastric juices or the acid chyme (broken-down food) because of its alkalinity.

# CHAPTER 2

## WHAT IS BILE REFLUX?

Bile reflux is a condition in which bile rises from the small intestine to the stomach through the pyloric valve. This valve is located in the lower part of the stomach, at its end, and generally opens just enough to release about one-eighth of an ounce (about 3.5 milliliters) of broken-down food at a time—not enough to allow bile or other digestive fluids to go up towards the stomach.

In normal digestion, food is digested in the stomach and then released into the small intestine through the pyloric valve.

In most cases, bile reflux occurs when the pyloric valve and the pylorus aren't adequately stimulated, mainly due to some sort of physiological problem. It's believed that a mechanical obstruction or some type of damage to the valve during surgery (for example, cholecystectomy) could also affect the functioning of the pyloric valve.

You already know that bile is a fluid your body uses mainly to break down fats. When you suffer from bile reflux, what you feel is not at all pleasant because this fluid rises from the small intestine to the stomach and/or esophagus. Many of us are familiar with this because it frequently coexists with the problem of acid reflux. In that case, gastric juices are able to ascend the esophagus and carry bile upwards. Both refluxes are not only very uncomfortable but can also lead to other complications if left untreated.

This digestive fluid irritates the stomach and leads to inflammation. It also damages the lining of the esophagus, causing it to become inflamed and potentially leading to a pre-cancerous disease called Barrett's esophagus. Both bile reflux and acid reflux can lead to these complications. However, unlike acid reflux, bile reflux is generally more difficult to control through simple lifestyle changes.

**The most common symptoms of bile reflux are:**

- Heartburn
- Abdominal pain
- Nausea
- Vomiting of bile
- Weight loss
- Cough or hoarseness
- Diarrhea

Bile and acid reflux often have similar symptoms, and it can be very difficult to determine which one is causing the discomfort or symptoms.

As I said before, bile is an alkaline substance and when it is mixed with the acid in our stomach, it results in a rash or an attack of burning and pain. Most people realize there's a problem when they experience a significant amount of heartburn—a burning sensation in the throat or chest that often includes a sour taste in the mouth.

**Complications of bile reflux can include:**

- Gastritis
- Gastroesophageal reflux disease (GERD)
- Ulcers
- Bleeding
- Damage to the esophagus (Barrett's esophagus)
- Cancers

Bile reflux is a problem that's often misdiagnosed because its symptoms are much like those of acid reflux. This is why many people who suffer from bile reflux are mistakenly diagnosed with gastroesophageal reflux, also known as GERD. The confusion isn't all that surprising, as bile reflux and gastroesophageal reflux share many symptoms.

Doctors often treat acid reflux with proton pump inhibitors, which, though they help alleviate symptoms, don't deal with the cause of the problem. (I'll talk about this later.)

A few bile reflux treatments are very effective; most doctors use the same medications to treat patients suffering from bile reflux and patients suffering from acid reflux. Unfortunately, this isn't very helpful because the true role of PPIs (proton pump inhibitors) is to inhibit the secretion of stomach acid in the stomach. For that reason, they aren't effective against bile reflux, since bile is produced in the liver (and not secreted by the parietal cells of the stomach). The only thing this type of medication can do to help a person suffering from bile reflux is alleviate heartburn caused by the presence of bile.

There are many reasons why bile travels up to the stomach. (This will be discussed in the next chapter.) The digestive system is configured as primarily a one-way passage through the body, with various valves and sphincters to ensure that food goes in only one direction. If these valves weaken or aren't stimulated properly, fluids could flow in the opposite direction, entering areas of the body where they can cause havoc and damage.

In the case of bile reflux, bile rises from the small intestine and irritates the mucosa of the stomach.

If the person also suffers from acid reflux (caused by weakness or relaxation of the lower esophageal sphincter), bile finds its way higher, severely irritating the lining of the esophagus and even the throat.

In addition to heartburn, the patient may experience choking or the feared Barrett's esophagus, which increases the risk of esophageal cancer. For that reason, it is so important that people who suffer from bile reflux gather as much information as possible about this problem, as well as the available treatment options.

Before starting any treatment, it's necessary to get a precise diagnosis. The easiest way to determine whether you suffer from bile reflux is through an endoscopy. With this test, your doctor can see if you have bile reflux, since the bile is visible to the naked eye. Your doctor will also be able to see whether there's inflammation in your esophagus or stomach, and may also take biopsies to rule out the presence of *Helicobacter pylori,* which can cause gastritis, ulcers and other complications.

It can be exasperating to not know which of these two conditions you are suffering from. For that reason, it's necessary to get the correct diagnosis. This is the first and most important step toward finding the right treatment.

If you've been diagnosed with GERD (gastroesophageal reflux disease) and your doctor's treatment doesn't seem to be working, it wouldn't be a bad idea to ask your doctor to double check for bile reflux disease so you can start on a path that gets you healthy once again.

## How Can You Determine the Difference Between Acid or Bile Reflux?

This is really difficult because, as I mentioned earlier, the symptoms of both refluxes are extremely similar. Sodium bicarbonate in water almost always provides immediate relief against acid reflux but it does absolutely nothing for bile reflux.

Sodium bicarbonate also releases carbon dioxide when it hits stomach acid, so it will likely cause belching almost immediately, though this effect depends on the amount of bicarbonate and acid in your stomach. Sodium bicarbonate doesn't cause such a reaction with bile. If you are unlucky enough to regurgitate stomach fluids, you will know the difference between bile and stomach acid. Bile is much more unpleasant!

# CHAPTER 3

# CAUSES OF BILE REFLUX

Before talking about what causes bile reflux, I want you to know that this is the part of the guide that I consider the most important because your treatment will depend on whatever is causing your reflux. That's why it is necessary to know that the causes of bile reflux (as well as the symptoms) may vary from person to person. Because of that, I will try to explain each of the possible causes of bile reflux.

- **Gallbladder surgery (cholecystectomy):** The liver uses the gallbladder to store bile, but sometimes the bile salts can get thicker and create stones in the gallbladder. This causes a lot of pain, and some people who experience it choose to have this surgery. Some experts claim that the pyloric valve may be damaged during this surgery.

- **Complications of gastric surgery:** Gallbladder surgery isn't the only type of surgery that can cause bile reflux. Other surgeries such as gastric bypass (for weight loss) and gastrectomy may also lead to this condition. The pyloric valve may be damaged during these procedures. As you know, this valve is responsible for allowing the food to enter the small intestine while not allowing bile to go up to the stomach. However, if this valve is weak or damaged due to any of the surgeries mentioned previously, bile reflux may occur.

- **Peptic ulcers:** This type of ulcer or lesion near the valve can block it and prevent it from closing or opening enough to allow the digested food to pass from the stomach into the small intestine. Thus, the stomach cannot empty as quickly as it should. The presence of stagnant food in the stomach can increase gastric pressure and cause bile reflux to the stomach and acid reflux into the esophagus.

**Other less-common causes:**

- **Pregnancy:** The changes that occur within the body during pregnancy have been known to cause temporary cases of bile and acid reflux.

- **Slow motility of the stomach:** Some people have bile reflux due to problems with gastric motility. In most cases, medications that increase motility (prokinetics) have been helpful in dealing with the problem.

- **Obesity:** An extreme weight gain can also lead to the development of bile reflux, though the effects can be reversed by weight loss.

- **Proton pump inhibitors:** This type of medication is frequently used to treat acid reflux, but there's information about and cases of people who have developed bile reflux after having taken this type of antacid for a long time.

- **Hypergastrinemia (excess gastrin levels in the blood):** It is a documented side effect of long-term use of proton pump inhibitors. Excessive levels of this hormone relax both the esophageal and pyloric sphincters. Interfering with acid production by taking this type of medication can be counterproductive because it can affect the biliary system, allowing bile to start flowing at the wrong time and to enter the stomach through a relaxed pyloric sphincter. However, acid production is part of a complicated biological feedback mechanism. This means that if you interfere with any mechanism of feedback, whether mechanical, electronic or biological, you can be sure that unexpected effects will result.

- **Gastrin deficiency:** Gastrin is a hormone secreted into the bloodstream by the stomach's G cells, which are stimulated by the presence of food in the gastric lumen. The main function of this hormone is to stimulate the production of stomach acid, but it also maintains the tone of the pyloric valve and increases the antral contractions around the pylorus, among other functions. Excessive levels or a lack/deficiency of this hormone can relax both the pyloric sphincter and the inferior esophageal sphincter, which can cause bile and acid reflux.

- **SIBO (small intestinal bacterial overgrowth):** The pressure of the gases caused by SIBO puts pressure on the gastrointestinal tract, causing bile reflux to the stomach. Some specialists theorize that when these gases try to leave, they can open the valves of the stomach and esophagus, moving the contents from the bottom up and causing burning. However, if the reflux exists independent of SIBO, the latter can make it worse.

- **Candida overgrowth (yeast):** There's a lot of information about how an overgrowth of this yeast in the intestines can cause "acid reflux", but not so much about whether it can cause bile reflux. Nevertheless, it's important that we know how it can lead to acid reflux and the theory about bile reflux.

  In most cases, problems begin when an accumulation of candida in the colon outweighs the beneficial bacteria that should be present in a healthy digestive tract. Food begins to ferment instead of decomposing and digesting. This fermentation produces excess gases that lead to swelling, belching and difficulty digesting food. The gases travel up the small intestine and stomach, and finally into the esophagus. When these gases manage to pass the esophageal sphincter, they carry with them stomach acid, which results in a burning or stinging in the chest.

  Candida overgrowth and SIBO can both affect gallbladder function. This is mainly because toxins produced by candida or SIBO are eliminated through the liver. With candida toxins in the body, the liver is constantly detoxifying the blood of the toxins that the candida produces. However, these toxins can acidify bile and cause bile acids to proliferate, making bile more irritating, corrosive and toxic. Toxic bile causes lesions and irritates tissues, such as the bile ducts, gallbladder and the sphincter of Oddi, which causes spasms and inflammation. When acid bile and pancreatic juices are mixed in the duodenum, they can create chaotic spasms and be thrown into the stomach, resulting in bile reflux.

• **Hypochlorhydria:** Low levels of stomach acid can cause the pylorus and pyloric valve to not be stimulated properly. This lack of stimulation causes premature shedding of the stomach contents into the duodenum, leading it to become irritated due to gastric secretions and chyme acid. It also causes the release of the hormones cholecystokinin and secretin into the bloodstream.

These hormones play important roles in the release of bile and pancreatic juices. For example, CCK (cholecystokinin) contracts the gallbladder to release all the bile accumulated in it and relaxes the sphincter of Oddi to allow bile to exit into the duodenum. On the other hand, secretin stimulates the pancreas to release pancreatic juices composed mainly of bicarbonate, water and pancreatic enzymes.

As you can see, in the end, what goes up to your stomach is not only bile, but also pancreatic juices and bicarbonate with bile, which alkalizes the acid chyme and the gastric secretions but in the wrong place (the stomach). Because the stomach doesn't have a defense mechanism against these agents, both bile and pancreatic enzymes irritate the stomach and make gastritis even worse.

And believe it or not, hypochlorhydria is one of the main causes of bile reflux and affects countless people throughout the world. Following, I'll talk about the most common causes of this problem.

## Main Causes of Hypochlorhydria

Different factors could lead to chronic low stomach acid, including anything that causes chronic stress in the body — poor nutrition, infections, poor relationships, poor posture and subluxation in the spine, constant worrying, fear and overuse of certain medications.

Although the production of stomach acid can increase with the use of supplements, doing so without looking for a possible underlying cause can result in aggravation of the symptoms. The following conditions and underlying factors should be checked first, as they are the most common causes of this problem.

- *Helicobacter pylori*: In many people, this bacterium inhabits the protective mucosal barrier that covers the stomach. (It's believed that it's present in approximately 50% of the population.) However, the excessive use of antibiotics, chronic stress, poor nutrition, etc. can alter or cause a change in the microbiota, decrease stomach acid production and cause an overgrowth of *H. pylori*. This bacterium inhibits the production of stomach acid by affecting the health of the parietal cells that produce the acid. As *Helicobacter pylori* overgrowth occurs, the bacterium produces an enzyme called "urease" that breaks down urea in the stomach into carbon dioxide and ammonia. This causes burps and halitosis (bad breath). It also neutralizes the acidifying effects of stomach acid, which enables the growth of *Helicobacter pylori* and places more stress on the gastrointestinal system. It affects the gastrointestinal lining and, in conjunction with life stressors and unhealthy eating habits, causes a multitude of chronic conditions.

- **Chronic stress:** Chronic stress alters the ability of the digestive system to produce HCL (hydrochloric acid) and other digestive juices. Our autonomic nervous system consists of two main branches: the sympathetic branch and the parasympathetic branch. Adequate digestion depends on our being in a parasympathetic dominant state. Chronic stress puts you in a sympathetic dominant state that restricts activity in the digestive tract and causes poor digestive function. When you're stressed, your body puts itself in a "fight or flight" state of alertness, which increases blood flow in your muscles, brain, heart and lungs and away from your digestive system. This is good if you are going to run away from a bear, but it is not if you are only going to have lunch. The "rest and digestion" mode allows you to carry out digestion properly.

- **Poor diet:** A diet rich in carbohydrates/processed foods, sugars, wheat, gluten, corn, soy, saturated fats, omega 6 fats, artificial sweeteners, GMOs (transgenic foods), etc. alters your microbiota, causes chronic inflammation, and increases the production of the stress hormone.

The stabilization of blood sugar is very important to normalize stress hormones. A low-carbohydrate diet high in rich-antioxidant and nutrient dense foods can help improve the levels of acid in your stomach.

- **Eating too fast or while in movement:** This is one of the biggest problems we have in our society. We eat lots of fast food and do so frequently throughout the day. It's extremely important to never eat when we are in sympathetic mode (fight or flight) and to take the time to relax, breathe deeply and increase parasympathetic activity. You must be relaxed for at least 15 minutes before eating and for up to one to two hours after finishing your meal. Also, chewing food well before swallowing is very important to facilitate the stomach's work.

- **Excessive use of antibiotics:** Antibiotics unbalance your microbiota and cause an increase in inflammation related to the intestine. This inflammation provokes an increase in stress hormones (cortisol, adrenaline, etc.), reducing the ability of the stomach to produce HCL.

- **Excessive use of NSAIDs:** In our society, we take nonsteroidal anti-inflammatory drugs (ibuprofen, naproxen, aspirin, etc.) as if they were candy. We believe that we will experience no serious problems if we take a relatively small dose each day. Unfortunately, this isn't true because NSAIDs irritate the lining of the stomach and reduce the ability of the stomach cells to produce stomach acid.

- **Proton pump inhibitors:** These types of drugs block the proton pumps (H+/K+ATPase) from the parietal cells so they don't produce hydrochloric acid. Unfortunately, because acid reflux is typically caused by hypochlorhydria, these drugs reduce stomach acid even more, leading to an excessive growth of microbiota and increased stress in the body. The histamine H2 receptor antagonists, also known as H2 blockers, also prevent histamine secretion by ECL (enterochromaffin-like) cells so that it cannot stimulate the parietal cells to produce stomach acid.

- **Small intestinal bacteria overgrowth:** It's not easy to say which comes first – low stomach acid allowing a high number of bacteria to enter the digestive system and proliferate due to undigested food particles (due to low levels of HCL), or SIBO (small intestinal bacteria overgrowth) causing chronic stress in the body, thereby reducing the ability to produce enough HCL. Either way, a huge connection exists between SIBO and low stomach acid.

- **Aging:** As we age, our systems slow down, especially the digestive physiology. This is even worse if we are stressing our body beyond its ability to adapt. If you start taking care of your body at an early age and keep your digestion at an optimal level throughout your life, you'll be able to keep producing enough HCL in later years. However, if you are over 50 years old, it's advisable that you pay attention to your stomach acid levels and consider treating deficiencies of vitamins and minerals (especially zinc and B vitamins). This could make a big difference in your body.

- **Food sensitivity:** Some of the most common food sensitivities cause significant stress in the body. Stay away from foods with gluten, corn, soy, peanuts and pasteurized dairy products. If you have sensitivities to many foods, it's a good sign that you have low stomach acid.

- **Mineral and vitamin deficiencies:** Zinc and B vitamins (particularly vitamin B3 [niacin]) are very important for the production of hydrochloric acid. Also, chloride, sodium and vitamins C, D and E are important for the optimal function of the epithelial cells of the stomach. However, deficiencies can cause a vicious cycle in which low stomach acid levels cause a malabsorption of certain vitamins and minerals necessary for the production of stomach acid. This happens because many vitamins and minerals are acid dependent or require a certain acidity to be ionized and absorbed.

- **Thyroid function:** Thyroid function can also influence the production of stomach acid. People with hypothyroidism produce less gastrin, the hormone that stimulates the parietal cells to produce hydrochloric acid in the stomach. A lack of necessary nutrients can also cause poor thyroid function. Re-establishing the necessary mineral capacity can address the issue, re-establishing the production of stomach acid.

- **Drinking liquids during meals:** Doing this dilutes the concentration of hydrochloric acid in the stomach (in total it represents 3-5% of the total gastric secretions), so your stomach will have to produce more acid (use more nutrients) to digest stagnant food in your stomach.

Other causes that I won't discuss here due to lack of information are the following: a vegetarian or vegan diet, candida overgrowth, and mitochondrial dysfunction/oxidative stress. Nor will I discuss the causes of achlorhydria, which is a more severe form of hypochlorhydria. Many of the factors mentioned here also cause achlorhydria, but there are others that are much more complex and severe.

The most accurate test to check for an HCL deficiency is the Heidelberg pH test, although this machine is not easy to find. (As far as I know, it is available only in some centers in the United States.) The easiest way to assess a HCL deficiency is to observe the levels of Co2 (carbon dioxide) and chloride in blood tests.

It can also work a mineral analysis of the hair. Jonathan Wright MD has identified that an HTMA is as accurate as the Heidelberg pH test.

If a HCL deficiency exists, it's very important to perform tests for *Helicobacter pylori*, parasites and other infections. If *H.Pylori* or other bacteria are present, this condition should be treated first. Otherwise, the treatment for the low stomach acid deficiency won't work.

It's important that you discard each of these possible causes because this problem can have a chain reaction of various causes; it's possible that one cause leads to another, and so on.

The objective is to attack the problem from the root cause. If you are not sure about some of the causes mentioned here, tell your doctor so you can work together. Through tests and lab work, you'll be able to determine what's causing your bile reflux.

Keep in mind that most doctors who practice conventional medicine are very focused on the disease itself and its symptoms, when the true focus should be on the particular patient. That's because each person is different and the cause of one person's illness may be different from that of another person. Because of this, a new concept in health care, known as "functional medicine," has grown in recent years. It is focused mainly on the patient and on identifying the cause of the chronic illness from which he or she is suffering instead of on treating only the symptoms of the disease or problem. Functional medicine also emphasizes the incorporation of nutritional solutions into the patient's lifestyle rather than simply offering drugs and surgical interventions. Therefore, it's advisable that you find a doctor who practices "functional medicine" to help you determine the cause of your problem.

No tests exist to determine some of these causes; that's the case with surgery, obesity and pregnancy. If you have had any of those surgeries or gone through any of those events, it's possible they are the cause of your reflux. Tests do exist for other causes. There's the Heidelberg pH test for hypochlorhydria, the hydrogen breath test for SIBO, various tests for gastric or intestinal motility, and the urine organic acids test for candida. Peptic ulcers can be confirmed through an endoscopy; I suppose that if your doctor did an endoscopy, he or she may have taken a look at your duodenum to determine whether you had a peptic ulcer.

# CHAPTER 4

# CONVENTIONAL TREATMENT FOR BILE REFLUX

Medication and lifestyle changes can be very effective at treating acid reflux, but they don't usually work as well with bile reflux. In the world of conventional or allopathic medicine, this condition can be treated in two ways: with medication or surgeries. But the truth is that there's no effective medication for bile reflux.

## Medications

- **Bile acid sequestrants:** Doctors often prescribe this type of sequestrant drug, which decreases the circulation of bile and removes bile acids from the digestive system. However, some studies indicate that these drugs are less effective than other treatments. The active component is cholestyramine.

- **Prokinetic agents:** These aid in the rapid emptying of the stomach and also tighten the lower esophageal sphincter. Long-term use of this medication can cause side effects such as fatigue, depression, anxiety and other neurological problems.

- **Sucralfate:** Its function is to bind to the hydrochloric acid in the stomach and form a barrier or protective layer over the stomach lining to protect it from acid, pepsin and bile salts. It also stimulates the production of prostaglandins by the mucosa and absorbs the bile salts.

- **Ursodeoxycholic acid:** This medication increases the flow of bile and decreases the amount of cholesterol in it. It also reduces the severity and frequency of the symptoms.

- **Proton pump inhibitors:** Doctors constantly prescribe this type of medication to block the production of acid in the stomach, but it isn't as effective against bile reflux. Plus, as I said before, there's information that indicates it can cause hypergastrinemia, thus aggravating bile reflux.

## Surgical Treatment

Doctors may recommend surgery if medications don't seem to be working for severe symptoms or if there are precancerous changes in the esophagus or stomach. Some types of surgeries may be more successful than others.

- **Diversion surgery (Roux-en-Y):** This procedure, which is also a type of surgery for weight loss, may be recommended for people who have had previous gastric surgeries in which the pylorus has been removed. In

Roux-en-Y, surgeons make a new connection in the small intestine to set apart the biliary drainage from the stomach and, thus, prevent bile from reaching the stomach.

- **Anti-reflux surgery (fundoplication):** In this procedure, the surgeons wrap and sew part of the stomach closer to the esophagus. This procedure strengthens the esophageal sphincter. Its goal is to prevent acid or bile reflux from reaching the esophagus.

# CHAPTER 5

# NATURAL TREATMENT FOR BILE REFLUX

[*Limitation of Liability: Before moving on, I want you to know that this is what worked for me. I cannot guarantee that it will also work for you because bile reflux happens for different reasons. It's possible that your cause is different from mine. But don't worry; if you have already visited your doctor and have received an accurate diagnosis, I believe this treatment can be of great help to you because it will help you treat and even eliminate some of your symptoms independently of what's causing your bile reflux. Besides, I don't think the treatment I followed could harm you because it is totally natural.*]

## What Can You Do to Get Rid of Bile Reflux?

Instantly getting rid of bile reflux seems impossible. However, once you know what's causing your problem, you can treat it more effectively and you will notice an improvement in less time. I discovered that my bile reflux was due to low stomach acid. As I explained in the chapter "causes of bile reflux", this causes the pyloric valve and pylorus to not be stimulated enough to work, or to shut down completely while digestion takes place.

I finally realized that the problem in my stomach consisted of two things: low stomach acid and the bile that irritated my stomach, worsening the former.

Let's start with the natural treatment that worked for me. I reduced to three simple steps the things I was going to do to treat my bile reflux:

1. Find the cause of my bile reflux and absorb the bile in my stomach.
2. Re-establish my natural levels of stomach acid.
3. Decrease my stress levels and release negative emotions.

Now let's look at these three steps in more detail. I'll try to make this as uncomplicated as I can with regards to the things you'll have to do and the supplements I will recommend that you take. This may cost you some money, but I can assure you that it will be better than paying for a medical appointment or buying expensive drugs that don't work. That's why I'm telling you that all these things will help you with more than just your bile reflux problem.

# FIRST STEP

## Find the Cause of Your Bile Reflux and Absorb the Bile in Your Stomach

In this first step, the first thing to do is find the cause of your bile reflux and absorb the bile in your stomach. For this, you must determine which of the possible causes mentioned in the chapter "Bile reflux causes" is triggering your reflux problems.

While you investigate the cause of your bile reflux, start absorbing the bile in your stomach. Basically, what you must do is create a "sponge" to absorb the bile in the stomach. For this you should make some changes in your diet. So, let's start with the diet.

The diet for bile reflux should be high in soluble fiber and low in fat. Soluble fiber helps absorb bile in the stomach, protect the stomach lining and increase intestinal transit. Here are some foods that contain a good amount of soluble fiber and that are recommended for gastritis due to bile reflux:

- **Cereals:** Oats, brown or white rice, barley, rye, quinoa, wheat bran and oat bran.

- **Vegetables:** Broccoli, brussels sprouts, beets, aubergines, artichokes, asparagus, carrots, lettuce, spinach, okra and cabbage.

- **Fruits:** Papaya, dragonfruit, bananas, pears, apples, strawberries, raspberries, blackberries, plums, blueberries and peaches. It is advisable you consume some of the acidic fruits mentioned above in smoothies made with almond milk. This will help neutralize their acidity.

- **Legumes:** Lentils, broad beans, peas, string beans or green beans, peas, chickpeas and soy.

- **Others:** Potatoes, green plantains, pumpkins, courgettes, and sweet potatoes.

You must include some of these foods in at least three of your main meals (breakfast, lunch and dinner) so that you can absorb as much bile as possible in your stomach. There are different types of soluble fiber, but pectin and mucilages are the most interesting because they trap bile acids and protect the stomach lining.

Mucilage appears in fruits like the fig and is very abundant in plants such as borage, plantain, purslane, mallow, marshmallow, marigold, violet, thought, hibiscus and nopal, in legumes such as green beans and fenugreek, and in lichens such as the Icelandic lichen or the Irish moss or carragen. Flax seeds or linseed are also very rich in mucilages, as are chia seeds and psyllium seeds. Agar-agar also contains mucilages.

The fiber pectin abounds in fruits and vegetables with great properties to prevent constipation. Apples and quince are very rich in pectin. Other foods rich in pectin include carrots, sweet potatoes, aubergines, pumpkins, figs, bananas, pears and plums.

A supplement that I highly recommend for its high content of soluble fiber is whole psyllium husk. This supplement absorbs and quickly removes the bile acids in the stomach. Psyllium husk helped me a lot in the moments when I had bile reflux attacks; if you really want to absorb as much bile as possible in your stomach, this supplement cannot be missed. My recommendation is that you take one or two teaspoons of this fiber in eight or 12 ounces of water, about two or three hours after eating lunch. Of course, make sure to drink plenty of WATER during the day and don't overdo it with the fiber, as the excess cannot be good.

## Protect Your Stomach

After you have started introducing some of the previously mentioned foods to your diet, it's time to start protecting your stomach. If you choose to take prescription drugs, the best thing your doctor can prescribe is a substance called sucralfate. This is quite harmless and may work for you. Its function is to bind to hydrochloric acid and create a protective layer on the stomach lining, although it can also absorb bile salts. Keep in mind that this is an antacid that acts on the stomach lining, so it is not recommended that you take it while you are treating low stomach acid. It can also cause constipation, so you should keep this in mind.

Another alternative that worked surprisingly well for me an infusion of nopal water and chamomile tea. Nopal's high mucilage content helps regenerate the stomach lining, as shown by several scientific studies.

My recommendation is that you cut several nopal cactus into small pieces and add water, then let it rest until it becomes thick or a slim consistency (about two or more hours). Half an hour before lunch and dinner, drink a cup of this water. For the chamomile tea, you can take a cup of it one hour before lunch and another cup one hour before dinner.

**Note:** *You can combine the nopal water with two or three tablespoons of aloe vera, which is rich in mucilaginous polysaccharides.*

# SECOND STEP

## Re-establish Your Natural Levels of Stomach Acid

After you start absorbing the excess bile in your stomach, it's time to normalize your stomach's pH levels. However, before you start doing this, it's important that you understand why you should have adequate acid levels in the stomach.

A healthy stomach must have a pH of between 1 and 2, and this is possible only by secreting the right amount of stomach acid. When a healthy stomach has a pH of 1-2, it secretes enough gastric mucus (which becomes part of the stomach lining) to help protect the stomach walls from stomach acid (which is very corrosive). The esophageal sphincter and pylorus are adequately stimulated, which helps prevent reflux into the esophagus and the premature emptying of the stomach contents into the duodenum. In addition, a healthy stomach's re-acidification time after being neutralized by the ingestion of food, beverages or alkaline solutions shouldn't exceed 20 minutes.

In a hypochlorhydric stomach, the production of stomach acid is low. Therefore, the stomach's contents are not acidic enough to initiate all the other digestive functions, but are acid enough to irritate the stomach lining, the duodenum and the esophagus.

Under this condition, the stomach doesn't stimulate an adequate production of gastric mucus, but its acidity is sufficient to irritate the stomach lining, which is now bare because of a lack of gastric mucus. This leads to a vicious cycle: the decrease in the production of hydrochloric acid causes a decrease in the production of the gastric mucus, which in turn causes irritation and can atrophies the cells that produce HCL.

There are many reasons why it's important to have good levels of stomach acid. Here are some reasons why stomach acid is important:

1. **Protection against infections:** A healthy stomach is sterile because the stomach acid kills bacteria, viruses and parasites. Insufficient stomach acid leads to the development of *H. Pylori, C. Diff,* fungi and parasites. Adequate levels of stomach acid also helps prevent small intestinal bacterial overgrowth (SIBO).

2. **Nutrient absorption:** If production of stomach acid is low, it could cause a deficiency of vitamin B12, amino acids, soluble vitamins such as A, D and E, and minerals such as calcium, iron, manganese, zinc and others.

3. **Digestion of proteins:** Stomach acid denatures animal protein and it's essential for converting pepsinogen into its active form, pepsin. This enzyme is responsible for the digestion of proteins. For its activation, pepsinogen must be exposed to a very acidic stomach pH.

4. **Communication of organs:** It alerts the pancreas to release pancreatic enzymes (amylase, protease and lipase) and the liver to produce bile—substances that are essential for the digestion of fats, proteins and carbohydrates. It also promotes the motility of the sphincter of Oddi and the small intestine and helps prevent gastroparesis. Although this really involves various hormones of the digestive system, a correct production of stomach acid enables this to be carried out with a better timing.

Now that you know a little more about the importance of maintaining good stomach acid levels, it's time that we get to the part where you'll learn how to naturally increase your levels of stomach acid.

Before starting, if you want to ensure that you have low production of stomach acid, I recommend doing the following test with baking soda.

## The Baking Soda Test

This test serves to approximate the levels of acidity in your stomach. Remember to perform this test on an empty stomach.

### Ingredients

- ½ glass of water (4 ounces)
- ¼ teaspoon of baking soda

Mix these two ingredients and take it on an empty stomach. Then take a clock or stopwatch and start timing until the first burp appears:

- 0-2 minutes - adequate amount of stomach acid
- 2-3 minutes - not enough stomach acid
- 3 or more minutes - stomach acid is very low, which could mean hypochlorhydria

I recommend performing this test for at least five days to get a better estimate of the amount of acid your stomach is producing.

## The Lemon Juice Test

When you are having stomach pain or heartburn, take a tablespoon of lemon juice. If this makes the pain go away, you are low in stomach acid. If the symptoms worsen, your stomach could be producing enough stomach acid.

## Another Test with Betaine HCl

This test consists of taking one capsule of betaine HCL and observing whether you feel a burning sensation during the first five to 15 minutes after your having ingested it. Betaine HCl is natural and extracted from beets. If you suffer from gastritis, the dosage of the capsule shouldn't be too high; otherwise, it could irritate your stomach lining. It would be better to do this test with capsules containing 200-350mg of betaine HCl.

To do this test, you must eat at least 15-20 grams of protein (approximately 80-100 grams of meat), either red meat or chicken breast.

Take the capsule with a little water during the middle of the meal and observe whether you experience any burning. If nothing happens and the symptoms improve slightly, the acidity decreases or the acid reflux goes away temporarily, you are low in stomach acid.

## Natural Treatment for Low Stomach Acid

To treat low stomach acid naturally, I recommend you to start with green juices at first. Following are two green juice recipes that helped me a lot while I was trying to get back my natural stomach acid levels. I want you to know that taking this juice will not only help you normalize the production of stomach acid, but will also decrease the inflammation and irritation in your stomach, detoxify and alkalize your body, nourish your cells, improve your digestion and give you more energy.

**NOTE:** *To make this green juice, you'll need an juice extractor. It's also preferable that the ingredients you use have been organically grown.*

My recommendation is that during the first week you start consuming the first recipe of green juices at morning (before breakfast). This is because it contains more ingredients than the second recipe and will therefore provide more nutrients, which itself will more quickly reduce the inflammation in your stomach and detoxify your body in a more effective way.

### 1- Green juice recipe (first week)

- 3 leaves of kale or spinach
- 1/2 cucumber
- 1/2 bunch of celery
- 1 green or yellow apple
- 3 medium carrots

### Directions:

Thoroughly wash each of these ingredients (mainly celery and kale or spinach). It's preferable that you peel the carrots. After you have thoroughly washed each ingredient put everything in the juice extractor. Once you get the extract, consume it quickly to prevent it from food oxidation (don't store it in the refrigerator).

### 2- Green juice recipe (second week)

- 1 bunch of celery

In this recipe, you will use only celery to make the green juice because, in fact, this pure celery juice will help you re-establish your levels of stomach acid.

Don't forget to drink this juice on an empty stomach and wait at least 20 or 30 minutes before breakfast. The amount of juice to drink is 16 ounces (500ml). Drink this every day for a month to notice results. Don't forget to protect and keep your stomach in constant recovery. For that you can drink chamomile tea and nopal water.

### Directions:

Wash each stalk and leaf under the tap, then put everything into the juice extractor. Drink the juice inmediately.

## Betaine HCl for Low Stomach Acid

Another very effective way to increase the production of stomach acid is to take capsules of betaine HCl. Note that when you suffer from gastritis, you cannot take high doses of betaine HCl, as too much betaine HCl could be very irritating for the stomach lining. It is recommended that you begin taking 200-350 mg capsules during a week or two with this dose. (The time may vary from person to person.)

At the end of these three steps I'll give you a list of recommendations and advice that I recommend you apply if you want to get better results when you do the things I explain in these steps.

It is important that while you're taking betaine HCL (if you decide to take it) you also take a good multivitamin and B complex supplement (containing the most common B vitamins), since B1 (thiamine), B3 (niacin) and B6 (pyridoxine) are required to produce stomach acid. Zinc is the mineral responsible for stimulating a catalytic enzyme called carbonic anhydrase. Without this enzyme, you cannot produce stomach acid. Sodium and chloride are also important; that's why it's advisable to replace table salt with another quality salt such as Himalayan or Celtic salt, as they provide not only chloride and sodium but also the trace elements and minerals necessary to carry out other functions within the body.

Don't forget that you should take the recommended daily dose of multivitamin and complex B along with Betaine HCL, since most minerals are acid-dependent; if they are not ionized by hydrochloric acid, they won't be absorbed or perform their functions within your body.

Another thing that can be of great help is including in your diet bitter herbs or foods (such as dandelion, gentian, fenugreek, ginger, spinach, kale, celery and green leafy vegetables) that stimulate the production of gastric juices.

Organic apple cider vinegar also helps increase stomach acid production. It is recommended that you take one or two tablespoons of vinegar with half a glass of water about 20-30 minutes before lunch and dinner. I have no experience with this but many people assure that it is very effective. If you are going to try it, keep in mind that if you are suffering from gastritis, it is not advisable to take any type of vinegar because acetic acid can be very irritating to the stomach lining.

While doing everything indicated in this second step, it is important that you protect your stomach. For this I recommend taking the nopal water and chamomile tea (as indicated in the first step) because it will help protect your stomach during the transition phase. During this phase, you may notice an increase in heartburn or burning symptoms in the stomach (which can be painful), but this usually lasts no longer than one or two weeks.

Those who don't have this information and who goes through the painful transition phase may think that it is better to abandon treatment. That's why I recommend taking the nopal water or chamomile tea to reduce the painful part of the transition phase.

# THIRD STEP

## Decrease Your Stress Levels and Release Emotions

In this last step, we will talk about what stress is, the damage it can cause in your body and what you can do to reduce it. We will also talk about emotions and how they can affect you physically and mentally.

## What is Stress?

Stress is a natural process of the human body. It is an automatic response to external conditions resulting in threats or challenges that require a mobilization of physical, mental and behavioral resources to face the problem.

The harmful effects of stress become apparent when you feel anger, anxiety or fear; these effects can include an altered heart rate, feelings of pressure in the chest and the loss of sleep or appetite.

Stress usually appears when part of the body makes a stronger-than-normal effort to face a difficulty (stressor). The other parts of the organism that give up their resources are harmed. Continuous stressful situations can be harmful over the long run.

The part of the nervous system that directs the body's resources to "fight or flight" is the sympathetic system and it's activated by adrenaline.

Stress causes an excess of adrenaline production and sympathetic activity. When stress is frequent, the body produces more than one hormone called cortisol.

If the situation persists for a long time, the body loses its capacity to produce cortisol and falls into extreme fatigue.

The part of the nervous system that directs the body's resources for mental processes, repair, maintenance, digestion and the rest is the parasympathetic system, which is activated by acetylcholine. A healthy nervous system keeps your sympathetic and parasympathetic activities balanced. Here are some primary stressors.

- **Emotional stressors:** anger, fear, rage, bad temper, sadness, frustration, grief/bereavement, among others.

- **Chemical stressors:** herbicides/pesticides, household cleaners, GMO foods, food additives and sugar, antibiotics/hormones, vaccinations, pharmaceutical drugs.

- **Structural stressors:** Overweight, excess exercise, an inadequate and prolonged working position.

Regardless of the source of stress, when it becomes chronic, it causes excessive activity in the sympathetic nervous system, excessive production of cortisol and a deficiency of activity in the parasympathetic nervous system. All this can result in dysfunction, disease, pain, discomfort, attention deficit, fatigue and loss of memory.

Let's look at an example. The hydrochloric acid you produce in the stomach is important for achieving good digestion. It destroys the microbes you take in along with your food. Its secretion results from the activity of the parasympathetic nervous system, but when you are stressed all the time, parasympathetic activity decreases, which also decreases the production of stomach acid and causes gastritis, reflux, fullness, malabsorption, irritable colon, immune disorders and inflammatory disorders.

Learning how to properly treat stress can be very helpful for your digestive system. Here are seven things you can do for decreasing stress:

1. **Practice meditation:** Find a quiet place away from distractions; clear your mind and concentrate on your breathing, between 10 and 20 minutes. Try to do this daily to give your body a physical and mental rest.

2. **Exercise:** Try to get in at least three hours of physical activity (walking, jogging or workout routines) a week. Physical activity is one of the best things you can do to manage the way you respond to stress.

3. **Listen to music:** Listening to a disc from your favorite artist or of relaxing sounds like waterfalls or noises from the rainforest or the sea may reduce and relieve tension.

4. **Perform yoga:** This discipline is quite useful when it's time to reduce tension; it involves controlled breathing, meditation and mental exercises.

5. **Write:** Keep a diary or write letters or emails to family or friends. Some researchers have shown that expressing oneself in writing can be a good way to reduce stress.

6. **Get a relaxing massage:** This therapy is one of the most pleasant and effective ways to reduce stress. There are different types of massages, including full body, shiatsu and stones.

7. **Rest well:** Sleeping the necessary number of hours daily is very important. Lack of sleep can decrease mental performance, resulting in a loss of concentration and a bad memory.

## Formula for Reducing Stress

To regain parasympathetic activity and get out of the vicious cycle of chronic stress, you need to consume the nutrients your body requires to produce acetylcholine.

There are many supplements on the market that are good for reducing/treating stress, but to promote the production of acetylcholine, it is advisable to take a supplement that contains the following nutrients:

- 800mg of choline
- 250mg of vitamin B5 (pantothenate)
- 20 mg of vitamin B3 (nicotinic acid)
- 40 mg of vitamin B1 (thiamine)
- 50 mg of manganese

The supplement doesn't have to contain the exact amount I have presented here but it should maintain a similar proportion. If you can't find a supplement with all those ingredients, you can buy complex B and choline separately and take it all together. Long-term consumption of a supplement with these ingredients is safe. Once you have reduced the stress in your life, you can take half the dose of each component of the formula for preventive purposes if you think it's necessary.

Another supplement I recommend as a natural alternative to antidepressants is an adaptogenic herb called *Rhodiola rosea*. This herb helps the body adapt to daily stress, and decreases anxiety, depression, fatigue and cortisol levels. You can get it online.

## What Are Emotions?

An emotion is an affective state that we experience, a subjective reaction to the environment that is accompanied by organic changes (physiological and endocrine) of innate origin, influenced by experience. Emotions have the function of adapting us to what surrounds us.

An emotion is also a process activated when the body detects some danger, threat or imbalance; the emotion puts in place the resources at its disposal to control the situation.

When you face a barrier or a difficulty in life, the emotion you experience at the moment, whether it's fear, anxiety, anger, boredom, interest, joy or enthusiasm, determines the type and amount of energy you are going to use to attempt to overcome the difficulty. The point of view from which you perceive the difficulty depends on your ability to overcome it and the mental state you're in at the moment. That's why the presence of the same difficulty can cause different emotions depending on your ability to overcome it. Being aware of this can help you produce interest in the problems that arise; this interest is the most appropriate and effective emotion for solving problems and overcoming difficulties.

**There are six basic categories of emotions**

Emotions are classified as positive or negative depending on their contribution to our well-being or discomfort. They all fulfill important functions for survival.

- **Fear:** We feel fear when we face a danger (real or imaginary). It allows us to avoid danger and act with caution.

- **Surprise:** We feel startled or astonished by a loud noise or an unexpected situation. It's a feeling that helps us orient ourselves into a new situation.

- **Aversion:** We feel disgust or revulsion at what we have in front of us. It produces rejection and we tend to walk away.

- **Anger:** It appears when things don't go as we want or when we feel threatened by something or someone. It is useful when it drives us to do something to solve a problem or change a difficult situation.

- **Joy:** We feel joy when we obtain something we desire or see an illusion fulfilled. It provides a pleasant feeling of well-being, safety and energy.

- **Sadness:** It appears when you lose something important or when you have been disappointed.

## This Condition Causes You Lots of Fear

At this moment, it's likely that your body is under greater stress, especially if you are suffering from pain. This not only boosts your stress levels, but also speeds up your "fight or flight" response. It probably adds to your fear, too, and I'll tell you something—fear is a big part of your healing process.

- You may be afraid that your condition could be something more serious.
- You may be afraid of never getting better.
- You may be afraid of not eating what you want again.
- You may be afraid of feeling bad when you're with friends.

Well, I can honestly say that you can improve. If the doctor hasn't found anything serious in your body, you are more likely to be successful with all the information I am giving you. So be patient.

Our bodies are like sponges; they absorb everything in our lives, including what we think about ourselves and some of the traumas that happen to us. However, if we don't free ourselves, what we absorb becomes "trapped" in our body. Then our bodies have to give us "pain" to get our attention.

**But, why do we feel pain?**

Because there's no other way to get our attention. Of course, some people are able to express their emotions or take the stress outside and break free of trauma but many of us don't; we keep it in there. The situation is like a pot filled with hot water; when it is full and gets too hot, it whistles (causes pain) to get our attention and let us know that something is happening.

This pain can manifest itself in various ways. It can come in the form of back or neck pain, irritable bowel syndrome, stomach problems such as reflux or gastritis, joint pain, headaches, panic attacks and many other diseases. Usually a doctor can determine, through tests and lab work, whether a problem exists in you body, but sometimes you still feel bad or in pain even when the doctor has found nothing. This could be a warning sign about something emotional going on inside of you. This isn't the case for everybody, but it is for many of us.

During this time of pain, you must start relaxing your body every day. This will help you release those emotions that may be lurking and silent within you.

I recommend that you do some of the seven things I suggested to reduce stress, primarily meditation or yoga. You don't really have to devote one hour a day; just 20 minutes of relaxation daily will be more than enough.

# CHAPTER 6

# GENERAL RECOMMENDATIONS

- Avoid drinking liquids with meals, as this dilutes the digestive juices and slows digestion.

- Decrease your consumption of sugar or sweet foods and refined carbohydrates.

- Raise the head of your bed about five or 10 inches.

- Chew food properly and eat it slowly.

- Eat small meals and split your large meals into five or six smaller ones throughout the day.

- Consume foods at room temperature; avoid those that are very cold or very hot.

- Prepare your food steamed, boiled or grilled.

- Don't take NSAIDs, aspirin or analgesics. If you need an analgesic, use paracetamol.

- Do some kind of physical activity daily. I recommend that you start walking for 15 or 20 minutes every day, preferably after eating, as this will help with the digestion process.

- Stay hydrated. Consume at least two liters of water daily.

- Reduce salt consumption and replace table salt for a better salt such as Himalayan or Celtic sea salt.

- Don't lie down after eating. Wait at least three hours after eating to go to sleep.

- Don't eat if you are stressed. Try to relax and get in a quiet atmosphere at lunch time.

- Consume foods with a soft consistency. Avoid raw or difficult-to-chew foods.

- Take note of foods that irritate your stomach lining, that you don't tolerate or to which you are allergic. These are the foods you should avoid for a while.

## Foods you should avoid:

- Avoid highly refined and processed foods, such as white flour products.

- Don't drink alcohol, energy drinks or caffeine-containingg drinks.

- Avoid tea (except for chamomile tea), coffee and carbonated drinks.

- Don't consume hydrogenated oils; replace them with coconut oil, olive oil or avocado oil.

- Avoid fried, fatty or spicy foods.

- Avoid dried fruits, raw fruits and vegetables, wheat bread, cookies, pasta and pickles.

- Some products and foods that also contain dairy are cheeses, ice cream, yogurt, custard, butter, whey protein, condensed milk, and milk-based desserts.

- Decrease your use of condiments and spices, such as garlic, onion, salt, cinnamon and clove.

## Foods you must include in your diet:

- Eat foods rich in flavonoids and antioxidants, such as vegetables as spinach, kale, broccoli, Brussels sprouts, celery, okra, artichokes, asparagus, green leafy vegetable and fruits as blueberries, strawberries, peaches, apricots, kiwi, mango, plums, Bosc and asian pears and red delicious apple. Vegetable juices such as carrot, beetroot and apple are a simple way to ensure an adequate intake of antioxidants that help fight the inflammation that causes gastritis.

- Increase your consumption of fish such as tilapia, trout, herring, wild salmon, cod, sardines, anchovies, small mackerel, flounder, haddock, hake, catfish, sole. Fish has anti-inflammatory effects and a high protein content with low reactivity.

- Include in your diet many fermented foods and probiotics that help reduce *Helicobacter pylori* (if you are infected), which can contribute to gastritis. These foods are sauerkraut, kefir, miso, tempeh, kombucha, kavas, sourdough and kimchi.

- Coconut water is an excellent choice to increase hydration. It cleans the body of inflammation and provides electrolytes. Coconut water isn't high in calories; however, you can use coconut milk/cream in your diet. This food provides nutritious fats and can help you maintain your weight.

- Choose an easily digestible protein powder such as hemp or sprouted rice grains, as these are easier to assimilate and should not aggravate gastritis. Avoid protein derived from whey, as it is made from dairy products and can cause an increase in your symptoms. Some sources of clean animal protein include grass-fed meat, organic eggs and organic chicken/turkey breast.

- Smoothies are a great way to nourish your body, especially when stomach problems compromise digestion; they are easier to digest and assimilate. You can combine fruits like papaya, banana, mango, peaches, pears, apples, melons or berries with a little almond butter and almond milk in a blender.

## Food Combining

It's important to combine food properly at meal time. This is true whether or not you suffer from a digestive problem, as combining food will allow you to attain optimal digestion and absorb the highest possible amount of nutrients. However, many people are unaware of the benefits of doing this, while others find it too complicated. In the long run, this bad habit can trigger digestive problems in those who are "healthy" people.

### Carbohydrates with protein

This is a rule that's rarely respected. We believe that for a meal to be "complete" it must have "everything" – a bit of carbohydrates, proteins and fats. Thinking that way leads us to err in a basic norm of conscious eating. The fewer ingredients in the same dish, the more nutritious and energizing the food will be.

If you're going to eat carbohydrates like rice, sweet potatoes or potatoes, it is best to combine them with vegetables. On the other hand, if you're going to eat proteins like chicken breast, turkey or fish, it is preferable that you combine it only with vegetables. These combinations of rice or potato (carbohydrates) with breast or meat (proteins) can slow down digestion and cause indigestion.

## Vegetables

Vegetables can be combined with each other with no problem. It is preferable to use the minimum of ingredients in the same food (four or five foods is enough) because ingesting a great variety of foods can slow down digestion.

## Fruits

It's advisable to avoid mixing watermelons, muskmelons and honeydews with other fruits. You can combine fruits of the same type – for example, sweet fruits with sweet fruits, acidic fruits with acidic fruits, and sub-acidic fruits and neutral fruits with any. Watermelon and melon should be eaten alone and not combined with other fruits. It's recommended that you always eat fruits on an empty stomach, before you consume any other food.

**Fats**

Excessive consumption of fats greatly slows down digestion and prevents the carbohydrates we consume from being absorbed quickly. This could wear down our pancreas and adrenal glands. In addition, excess fat can lessen blood flow, which has its own serious repercussions, like chronic fatigue, heart problems, hormonal imbalance, diabetes or prediabetes, and obesity.

Foods that are high in fat include all animal foods, oils, nuts, seeds, avocados, and coconuts. If you're going to eat foods high in fat, ideally you should do so at the end of the day so that you don't slow down the digestion of other foods you eat during the day.

## Supplements for Gastritis

- **Licorice:** This is the root of the plant Glycyrrhiza glabra and is known for its antispasmodic and anti-inflammatory properties on the stomach lining, which helps treat stomach heaviness, indigestion and flatulence. Licorice root contains glycyrrhizin, which is a substance that can cause hypertension, so it is recommended that you use licorice root free of glycyrrhizin, known as DGL. Take one to three chewable tablets at a dose of 300-400 mg per tablet, about 20-30 minutes before eating, three times daily.

- **L-Glutamine:** This is the most abundant amino acid in the body. It's necessary to helps repair damaged tissues. Glutamine can help decrease inflammation of the stomach and damage caused by *Helicobacter pylori*. Take five to 10 grams of glutamine daily (divided into two intakes) on an empty stomach.

- **Probiotics:** Opportunistic bacteria such as *Helicobacter pylori* can damage and cause problems in the digestive tract. That's why probiotics are necessary – they help increase beneficial organisms in the digestive tract. Consider taking a probiotic supplement with at least 10 billion CFUs. You can also include probiotic drinks like kefir and kombucha.

- **Slippery elm:** This is the inner bark of the elm or Ulmus rubra. It has some of the same effects as the mucilages of the marshmallow root. The content of the mucilage of the slippery elm can be very beneficial in people suffering from gastritis, as it helps soften the gastrointestinal tract and it absorbs bile acids from bile. Take two capsules three times a day or, if in powder form, mix one teaspoon in a glass of water, juice or tea.

- **Aloe vera:** This plant is rich in mucilages that help protect the stomach lining and cover the gastric mucosa. It is also known for its anti-inflammatory and regenerative properties, which is very useful in cases of gastritis or stomach ulcers. Chew two to three tablespoons of the aloe vera gel, preferably on an empty stomach.

- **Gamma-oryzanol:** This supplement is obtained from rice bran, which is found in the germ and bran of this plant. Gamma-oryzanol is a complex formed by a mixture of plant sterols and ferulic acid. It helps protect the stomach lining, so it is indicated for cases of gastritis and ulcers. Take 100 mg of gamma-oryzanol three times a day for three to six weeks.

- **Zinc:** This mineral is necessary to stimulate a catalytic enzyme called carbonic anhydrase, which is found inside parietal cells. Without this enzyme, stomach acid and bicarbonate cannot be produced. Without zinc, this enzyme is not stimulated and cannot catalyze $H_2O$ (water) and $CO_2$ (carbon dioxide) in the $HCO_3$ ions (bicarbonate) and $H+$ (hydrogen) that form the stomach acid. The bicarbonate acts as a buffer against stomach acid so that it doesn't irritate the stomach lining. It is important to keep a zinc-to-copper ratio of 15:1 or 10:1. Take 30 mg of zinc and 2 mg of copper with food once a day. Consult a doctor before using this supplement.

- **Zinc carnosine:** This is a complex of zinc and the amino acid L-carnosine, which is also a potent antioxidant. This supplement helps protect the stomach lining from opportunistic bacteria such as *Helicobacter pylori* and from damage caused by NSAIDs (nonsteroidal anti-inflammatory drugs). It also supports the health of gastric cells. Take two capsules (75 mg) twice a day for about eight weeks.

Also consider taking a good supplement of B vitamins and other vitamins such as A and E. B vitamins are necessary for the proper functioning of the body; they also help obtain energy from the food you eat. Vitamin A helps with tissue repair and vitamin E is a potent antioxidant that fights free radicals. Both vitamin A and E are fat-soluble and have a cumulative effect on the body, so it's advisable to not abuse these supplements or to consult a doctor before you begin the supplementation.

# CONCLUSION

We've reached the end of this book, where the only thing missing is for YOU to take action. The first thing to do is find the cause of your bile reflux. While doing that, you must absorb the excess bile in your stomach. For this, you must introduce to your diet some of the foods I mentioned in the first step. You must also introduce a supplement high in soluble fiber, like psyllium husk, to absorb more bile in the stomach and to protect the stomach with some of the natural options I mentioned.

> **IMPORTANT:** If you're taking antacids, it is not advisable to continue with the second step of the treatment, as this type of medication will inhibit the production of stomach acid, which could be counterproductive. It is recommended that you not consume any antacid medication while you perform this treatment.

Following this, you will have to treat the low stomach acid. For this, you must start consuming the first type of green juice during the first week and the second type of green juice (this is the most important one) during the second week. If after consuming the green juice you feel only a slight improvement, I recommend that you follow the protocol with betaine hydrochloride and take a good multivitamin or zinc carnosine and B complex.

In this step, it's extremely important that you be strict about some of the things I suggested to protect your stomach. This is because you will be stimulating the production of stomach acid, which can be irritating and painful.

The idea is to keep the stomach lining in constant recovery while normalizing the production of stomach acid, which in turn will help the stomach regain its ability to produce a sufficient amount of gastric mucus.

In the third step, you should begin reducing stress and working on your emotions. Take some time for this because it is as important as the first two steps. If you skip this step, you will be making the recovery of your stomach more difficult.

Once you try some of the things I've recommended, you can make the necessary changes and adjustments and stick with what works best for you. I really believe that if you do all the things I mentioned in this guide, you'll start to notice improvement in less than two weeks. Just be consistent and patient.

Don't forget that before starting any treatment you should visit your doctor. This way you'll ensure that you have no serious problems that may require another type of treatment.

I wish you the best in life and I hope you get well soon.

Paul Higgins

# ABOUT THE AUTHOR

**Paul Higgins** is an avid health researcher and author of various books about different digestive disorders. He was diagnosed with bile reflux, acid reflux, chronic gastritis, and other digestive problems —such as dysbiosis and leaky gut— in early 2013.

During the course of about four years, he researched everything he could find about bile reflux, gastritis and the other digestive problems he was suffering. He learned how the digestive system works (including the physiology of gastrointestinal secretions), as well as how and why common digestive problems such as acid reflux, bile reflux and gastritis occur. He managed to heal his digestive problems through a therapeutic strategy with a holistic medical approach different from what conventional medicine offered him.

Now, this author of books helps other people who are also going through the same situation that he once went through. Through his books, Paul shares all the information, knowledge, and experience acquired over his four years of research on gastritis, acid and bile reflux, and other digestive problems.

ALSO BY PAUL HIGGINS:

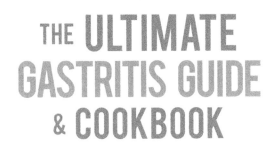

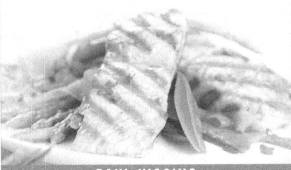

Made in the USA
Las Vegas, NV
06 March 2025

19165444R00046